AROMATHERAPY

A Comprehensive Guide To Get Started With Essential Oils

JESSICA THOMPSON

© Copyright 2018 by Jessica Thompson

All rights reserved.

The following eBook is reproduced below with the goal of providing information that is as accurate and reliable as possible. Regardless, purchasing this eBook can be seen as consent to the fact that both the publisher and the author of this book are in no way experts on the topics discussed within and that any recommendations or suggestions that are made herein are for entertainment purposes only. Professionals should be consulted as needed prior to undertaking any of the action endorsed herein.

This declaration is deemed fair and valid by both the American Bar Association and the Committee of Publishers Association and is legally binding throughout the United States.

Furthermore, the transmission, duplication or reproduction of any of the following work including specific information will be considered an illegal act irrespective of if it is done electronically or in print. This extends to creating a secondary or tertiary copy of the work or a recorded copy and is only allowed with an expressed written consent from the Publisher. All additional rights reserved.

The information in the following pages is broadly considered to be truthful and accurate account of facts, and as such any inattention, use or misuse of the information in question by the reader will render any resulting actions solely under their purview. There are no scenarios in which the publisher or the original author of this work can be in any fashion deemed liable for any hardship or damages that may befall them after undertaking information described herein.

Additionally, the information in the following pages is intended only for informational purposes and should thus be thought of as universal. As befitting its nature, it is presented without assurance regarding its prolonged validity or interim quality. Trademarks that are mentioned are done without written consent and can in no way be considered an endorsement from the trademark holder.

DISCLAIMER

*This information is for reference purposes only.
Statements are not intended as a substitute for professional healthcare nor meant to diagnose, treat, cure or prevent medical conditions or disease.
Every illness or injury requires supervision by a medical doctor or an alternative medicine practitioner.*

CONTENTS

1 HISTORY AND TRADITION..6

2 AROMATHERAPY & ESSENTIAL OILS DECODED..............10

3 ESSENTIAL OILS BUYING GUIDE...18

4 WAYS TO USE ESSENTIAL OILS..22

5 GENERAL SAFETY PRECAUTIONS..26

6 TWELVE ESSENTIAL OIL RELAXANTS.................................28

7 THE BASIC ESSENTIAL OILS...38

1
HISTORY AND TRADITION

Plants are not only incredible sources of nutrients and foods for man, present in them are also many of nature's wondrous components that have extremely been helpful in solving man's most challenging health conditions. Plants contain numerous phytonutrients which and among other things, include a plethora of extracts that have a phenomenal aromatic essence, for example essential oils. Sometimes dubbed the "soul" of plants, essential oils have long been a mainstay in many culinary and therapeutic preparations. In contrast to its name, essential oils don't typically present as oils from the outside; they appear more watery, and so less viscous than would be expected of oils. That said, essential oils are extremely volatile and highly concentrated, and so are usually laden with a wide range of organic components.

Vitamins, hormone and certain chemicals fall into the group of essential oils needed by plants to successfully carry out life functions. For example, flowers have essences that help them attract plants, and this is vitally important for their pollination. In shrub trees, resin is the essential oil that helps to heal wounds faster while providing enough resistance when extremes of weather set in. Essential oils help to keep the plant moist by preventing excessive water evaporation. But that's not all, they can also help plants to ward off predatory attacks by serving as a deterrent to external aggressors while communicating the danger to nearby plants and trees.

Due to their wide range of components and aesthetic presence, essential oils have long been used by man in the preparation of air fresheners, as food enrichment and also medically, to heal the body of many conditions.

The medical use of essential oils dates back to thousands of years ago where they were included in the practice of aromatherapy. Shen Nung, a Legendary Chinese ruler, is credited with the initial efforts that brought the medicinal properties of plants to fore. He wrote 'Pen Tsao' (c. 2700-3000 BC) - the first written herbal text that contained over two hundred botanicals. His initial findings sparked curiosity among archaeologists and scientists alike, making civilizations in China, the Middle East and India explore the therapeutic benefits of essential oils during these early periods. For example, a traditional Hindu form of healing called Ayurveda is synonymous with the use of local herbs in the treatment of many conditions.

In Ancient Egypt, waters, incense, resins and ointments were extensively used in religious ceremonies. It is also believed that Queen Cleopatra also had massive collections of flowers in her garden, and used the essences obtained therefrom for perfuming herself and surroundings. Pharaohs were strongly linked with the use of Terra cotta urns. And in Rome, soldiers found the magical benefits of honey and used it alongside myrrh to heal wounds. Roman emperors fancied perfumed baths as it gave the much-needed relaxation and soothing feeling. Both Old and New Testaments of the Bible also contain recipes that had aromatic compounds in their preparation.

In Europe, widespread exploration and use of essential oils were facilitated in the 16th century when glass distillation methods were discovered. More robust trade routes and the invention of the microscope meant bioactive compounds could also be better studied. Hence, extraction of plant essential oils became popular in plants like Italian chamomile, French rosemary and English lavender. Queen Elizabeth I is known to have used an overwhelming supply of English lavender oil during the course of her reign, and the tradition was continued throughout the 64-year rule of Queen Victoria.

The early 20th century brought aromatherapy to life in modern history as French chemist Rene-Maurice Gattesfosse who, inadvertently, set his arm ablaze in the laboratory was relieved after dipping his hands in the closest vat of cold liquid, coincidentally lavender oil. While previous injuries from chemical burns brought extended and deep pains, blisters, inflammation induced redness and scarring, Gattesfosse's burn surprisingly didn't present similar problems, with only slight pains and no scarring. It was obvious this had something to do with the lavender oil, and so reckoned Gattefosse too. This intriguing observation led him to coin 'aromatherapy,' a word he used to describe the exceptional healing he had received.

But he wasn't going to let the knowledge of lavender oil go down the drain, and so he dedicated many more years in the research of the attendant health benefits of essentials which culminated in his well-known book "Aromatherapy" that was published in 1937. In it, Gattefosse stated his findings on essential oils, and consequently further brought the medical use of these agents to limelight. With the book becoming a staple in the collections of essential oil enthusiasts, the work was translated into English in 1993. Unsurprisingly, the second edition is still available in print after 70 years.

Gattefosse efforts meant other scientists like Jean Valnet, a French physician, delved deeper into essential oils. Valnet chose to use essential oils in helping heal wounds during World War II. Soldiers that would have otherwise been amputated were able to successfully manage their injuries by getting treated with essential oils. Jean's book 'The Practice of Aromatherapy' further advanced the cause of essential oils as it made the oils become widely accepted, ensuring they were adopted for medical and psychiatric use in France in the 1960s. Marguerite Maury published more discoveries on essential oils in 1962, and so these oils gradually became mainstream ingredients in the cosmetic industry. Robert Tisserand's 'The Art of Aromatherapy' provided the springboard for the popularity of aromatherapy and massage, propelling them to become a common practice throughout the United Kingdom and the United States.

The popularity of aromatherapy, as it gradually spread to other parts of the world, coupled with the dynamic rise of natural medicines in the 1980s ensured its reliability as a health regimen which has since gone on to become a veritable way of treating many health conditions. So much so that in 2008, it accounted for about 95% of the world's essential oils market, translating to close to US$ 4.6-billion. The aromatherapy industry has consistently grown ever since at the rate of 7.5% annually over the last decade, and the trend may not go down south anytime soon with everyone getting on board to have a feel of the unrivaled natural healing experience.

2
AROMATHERAPY & ESSENTIAL OILS DECODED

First off, aromatherapy is not supposed to be a one-size-fits-all substitute for all conditions where traditional medical treatment is intended. While its activity has been well documented, aromatherapy is only an extension of a long-running practice involving the use of plants to treat medical conditions. For example, the aspirin we use today was a product of experiments conducted at the Bayer & Co dye factory using a byproduct obtained from the spirea plant.

Chemist Felix Hoffman is credited with synthesizing the first known acetylsalicylic acid which had earlier been known to be helpful in the treatment of rheumatism. Cold colds are a common bane, but we've also been able to successfully remedy the condition using Vicks Vaporub whose active ingredients are synthetic forms of many products including laurel tree i.e camphor, mint (menthol), and eucalyptus as well as nutmeg, cedar leaf and pine oils. Coca-Cola was initially marketed as a product that served as a 'nerve tonic,' with ingredients including essential oils of spices and citrus fruits.

Aromatherapy is interestingly an amazing science, but it is also an art, making it an exhilarating but equally daunting task when studying the nitty-gritty of its wide scope. On the whole, essential oils are a group of aromatic molecules gotten from plant part and materials like leaves, petals, needles, twigs, seeds, resin, wood and rind. Here are basic concepts and terms to easily understand the nuances of the pharmacological and botanical data in the study of Aromatherapy.

ABSOLUTE OILS

Absolute oils are the semi-liquid or alcohol soluble oils gotten from plants with a solvent extraction process that produces very low yield. For example, a thousand pounds of flowers yield only about one teaspoon of jasmine absolute. A teaspoon of "rose absolute" can be gotten from around five thousand pounds of petals. With distillation, however, an equal amount of ottor (attar), a rose essential oil requires a staggering ten thousand pounds of petals. Hence, rose otto costs expectedly twice as much the price of rose absolute regarded to be among the most expensive essential oils.

BLENDED OILS

Blended oils are essentially a recipe or formula that is derived from synergizing or combining a host of essential oils. The selection of blended oils is literally unlimited with more than enough options abound. Expert aromatherapists also have their own preferred combinations or recipes usually advised by their extensive knowledge and experience.

While going with blends comes across as a great way to experiment with pre-combined formulas, it may however be time-consuming, so learning the essential oils and putting ideas into practice is a trusty way of getting a reliable mix for any medical condition or purpose. Thus, blended remedies may appear as having the same ingredient composition, however, they will almost always not be combined in the same proportion.

CARRIER OIL

Essentials oils are characteristically thin and watery, but even if they are unusually thick, there's little to no chance of having them dissolve in water. Essential oils are only exceedingly soluble in alcohol or fatty oils. Carrier oils are used to dilute essential oils, and are sometimes referred to as base oil. They include products from a number of sources like nuts, seeds, trees or vegetables. Popular carrier oils are those of coconut, almond, sunflower and jojoba.

Blends of essential oils are usually composed of a carrier oil combined with minute quantities of essentials since essential oils on their own are noticeably too harsh to be used when not diluted, or too costly to be used without a carrier oil. However, a few of these oils can be used as carrier oils, examples of which include tea tree or lavender. Apart from making for more seamless application, carrier oils are great for keeping the moisture of essential oils on the skin for extended periods. Besides, diluted essential oils are long lasting as only small quantities are needed during the massage process.

EXTRACTION

The term "Extraction" refers to the process of obtaining oil molecules stored in plants. Understanding the extraction process is key to knowing the inherent properties of an oil. It also tells more about its benefits as well as ways to purchase and use. Extraction of oil molecules from plants can be carried out in many ways. These include steam or water distillation, expression, or by solvent extraction.

- **Steam or Water Distillation**
  Steam distillation using pressure remains one of the most efficient processes of extraction. Here, the plant is heated, and as formed vapor cools, essential oil is what is obtained. On the other hand, water distillation involves covering the plant material in water and subsequently heating up the plant. Distillation by water takes a longer time to go to completion, and therefore comes with the risk of losing essential oil components that are not overly resistant to heat, making steam distillation the more preferred extraction method.
- **Solvent extraction**
  This process of extraction is a great alternative when sensitive parts like jasmine and rose petals are the source of essential oil. Solvent extraction ends a method known as enfleurage where glass placed petals are covered with an odorless fat or oil. On the alternative, flowers can be stirred into heated oil. A "pomade" or "concrete" is formed when enough flowers

have saturated the oil or fat. The pomade formed afterward is soaked in alcohol to absorb the fragrance produced by the fat, and the two are then separated. As the alcohol evaporates, the particulate plant matter is left behind. This is what is referred to as the flower's "absolute" essence. The fat is used in the manufacturing of soap. If benzene, hexane, or other synthetic petrochemical is used as a solvent, the "absolute" essence gotten from the process comes with fewer benefits than alcohol - a sugar derived organic substance.

- **Expression**
  This is used for oil extraction from the rind of lemon, bergamot, orange or other citrus fruits. While expression used to be considered a laborious process that could only be done manually using the hands, the advent of savvy technology processes have ensured expression of rinds is now a mechanized process. For home practice, you may experiment with a fruit rind by cutting off a peel segment of washed and dried fruit and pierce this peel with a knife tip. Place over a bowl and carefully squeeze the rind to get drops of essential oil. Preserve your oil by storing in a dark glass bottle and keep in a cool place. This may seem a crude way, but your product is just as fine as any commercially sold essential oil obtained from citrus, and so can be a reliable product when you need to perform aromatherapy.

In a process recently discovered, carbon dioxide carbon dioxide can also be used at low temperatures for the extraction process, resulting in highly fragrant aromas. Although preferable to solvent extraction, the only caveat with this process, aromatherapists believe, is in the fact that it requires the use of highly expensive equipment to carry out the extraction process successfully. Consequently, the oils obtained are more expensive and may not be easily within reach. Others at dissent with this process say the temperature required for CO_2 extraction is barely high enough for proper distillation of the plant molecules. Hence the essential oils obtained, they posit, should not be used for therapeutic purposes but rather in candles, soaps and room deodorizers.

5% OR 10% OILS

These blends are often associated with costly essential oils, although suppliers ensure they are budget friendly by using career oil to dilute them. It is noteworthy, however, that the stipulated percentage is not to mean the quality of essential oil but its quantity. Hence when bottles are described as containing '5% Rose Absolute in Jojoba,' this means that the bottle contains 95% jojoba oil combined with 30 drops of 1.5ml of pure rose absolute.

FRAGRANCE & PERFUME OILS

Fragrance and perfume oils are synthetically made aromas designed to simulate natural aromas but they are dissimilar to pure essential oils. The scents of fragrance and perfume oils mimic natural scents, bringing qualities of richness, familiarity, endurance and complexity. However, these fragrances are chiefly made to be combined with soaps, perfumes, skincare and hair products as well as in making candles, household cleansers and deodorizers. They are never designed for use in aromatherapy. Common examples of these oils are Black Rose, China Rain, Forest, Vanilla and Lily of the Valley.

HYDROSOLS

Also referred to as hydrolat or flower/floral water, hydrosols are the vapor by-product obtained after a distillation process. They essentially have the same fragrance and benefits of essential oils, and they are usually employed in the making of skin care products that have essential oils. Cosmetically intended flower waters include those made from neroli, chamomile and rose petals.

NEAT

Due to the strong concentration of essentials and the high chance of hurting the skin if applied directly, most essentials come with the warning "Do not apply neat." But there are few exceptions; tea tree and lavender oils can be applied to the skin directly when in combination with career oils.

ORGANIC OILS

Organic essentials are those produced from plants that have not been subjected to synthetic applications or processes. There is often a USDA green and white circular seal on food products certified to be organic; the same seal goes on "organic essential oils." Hence if pesticides and synthetic fertilizers were used on a plant or the plant was processed artificially and has chemical preservatives or additives, the essential oil derived therefrom will not come across as organic.

"Organic" might loosely be connected with words like "chemical-free," "no pesticides," "100% natural," "grown wild," and "all-herbal" among others. However, they are not always to mean they are truly 100% organic. A best practice to ensure safety and authenticity is to look out for the USDA seal on the product or be convinced that the dealer is truly letting you have an organically grown and manufactured product.

Two contrasting groups exist in aromatherapy as regards the superior aroma and benefit, or otherwise, of organic essentials as opposed to non-organic oils. While some believe that essential oils are laden with a significant contaminant load due to being highly concentrated (no substantial scientific backing to this claim though), others hold that an effectively carried out distillation process leaves out any fertilizer or pesticide contaminant and ensures the water, steam or alcohol distilled oils are essentially pure products. The choice of organic oil over non-organic alternatives is absolutely a personal decision. Nonetheless, the immense natural composition and benefits make organic oils get the nod for use in aromatherapy. The only caveat being that they are always more expensive, and probably twice as much, when compared to non-organic options.

How to Choose Essential Oils

As with many popular products, choosing the right essential can be a mazy decision, complicated by the presence of many options and varieties. There are also oodles of fragrances to choose from when looking to douse stress, improve your mood or use for health purposes. The extracts vary in purpose too, due to their components, and so while some are best used as topical creams for reversing scars and acne symptoms, others are first choice stress relievers.

Whatever your reason for cashing in on an essential oil, ensuring that the scent is very appealing is a basic thing to look out for; some essential oils can present pungent smells while others, like those made from citrus, are characteristically flowery in smell. You also want to keep the products some good distance away to prevent triggering reactions like headache; this is especially important if the essential is undiluted. Taking a break in between tests will also help make better decisions as over saturation of smells can impair your judgment of the scents.

Another tripwire to look out for is if your retailer sets a specific price for all essential oils. Considering the fact that some essential oils aren't common and so should be expectedly expensive, stacking essential oils at the same price may be a subtle sign that some of the oils, especially the rare ones, are not original. For example, they may have been subjected to cheaper distillation methods or have undesired by-products in the product packaging.

If oily solvents tend to present challenges or trigger allergic responses, you may consider not going with essential oils diluted using vegetable oil since chances exist of having residues in the final product. A nifty way to go about detecting if your essential was diluted using vegetable oil is to place a tiny drop of it on a paper. If residues are left behind as the drop slides off, you likely have a vegetable oil diluted with essential oil.

Top quality essential oils are excellently pure and shouldn't portend any allergic reactions or dangers when used. Pure essential oils are also first choice for aromatherapists since they are clearly stronger in therapeutic effect than synthetic oils. Essential oils should also stored properly in a dark or navy blue container as this will help to preserve the ingredients. Exposing your product to sun lights sets the recipe for product deterioration and, consequently, loss of activity when used for therapeutic purposes.

3
ESSENTIAL OILS BUYING GUIDE

TOP 10 LISTS

It is believed that over 3000 essential oils exist, and of these, about 300 are therapeutically relevant and routinely used in aromatherapy. Out of these therapeutically beneficially oils, 101 are traded globally. In most cases, every merchant, manufacturer or practitioner has varying "top ten" lists of essential oils, and they are never the same since there are varying determinants to be factored. For example, you may have a "Top 10 Best Selling, " Top 10 Florals," and "Top 10 Recommend" lists of essential oils. So you may decide to go with your own list of Top 10 essential oils based on the needed criteria.

CHOOSING ESSENTIAL OILS

The categorization of essential oils can be done in a number of ways. While some are alphabetical, others may be labeled botanically, chemically, aromatically, according to ailment or some other sort of categorization. There are either positive or negative states for the physical, emotional and mental wellbeing of an individual. And hence, reversing any unwanted health condition demands an equally potent solution. Essential oils can be labeled as positive or negative in effect, depending on their effect. "Negative" essential oils are calming, relaxing, and sedative or essentially tension reliving in nature. Positive essential oils, on the other hand, are meant to invigorate, rejuvenate, or stimulate the body for a better mood. This method has been used in chapters 6 and 7 to give a list of 24 basic essential oils, all of which are top oils recommended by retailers, aromatherapists, authors and manufacturers.

However, the list is obviously not exhaustive and there are surely many more essential oils you may include, depending on your intended use. The given list is only a good reference point when getting started. Select five oils from the list of "12 Essential Oil Relaxants" and another five from the list of "12 Essential oil stimulants" as may be defined by the condition or use. With that out of the way, visit a store where essential oils can be sniffed and have a feel of the options you want. Anything off is not what you want, so discard such aromas and go for oils that are appealing to your sense of smell. Your essential oils list can be grown in due course as you get to know more about them or based on future needs.

LABELING

Been abreast of labeling when choosing a product, and more so when buying an essential oil, can be a goldmine. Manufacturers may not intentionally be deceptive, but essential oils can be labeled in different ways, making it difficult to identify what option you should go with. You don't necessarily need to be a pro as regards essential oils, but there are a few things to look out for in the labeling before choosing one.

STRAIGHT-FORWARD LABELING:

- Therapeutic Essential Oil
- 100% Pure Essential Oil
- No additives, no pesticides
- First distillation
- Maximum therapeutic benefit
- Undiluted & pure

You may not have the most acute awareness of the nuances in essential oil labeling. However, getting to know the basics can save you time and money when buying a product. For example, a product containing only three drops of lavender oil in 8 ounces of jojoba oil may be labeled as "100% pure essential oil," and that may not be faulted if the product wasn't marketed as "undiluted." First distillations are likely going to be the highest quality you can get, with subsequent distillations being essential oils that are slightly weaker.

DUBIOUS LABELING:

- Rich in essential oil
- Vitamin-enriched oil
- Blend containing pure essential oil
- Extracted from whole plant
- Plant-based oil

Also important in the labeling of essential oils is checking for the plant part that the oil was obtained from. For example, if research establishes that the best essential oil of a plant is only obtainable from its roots, going for a product that contains the "leaf extract" of such plant may not be a great idea. Essential oil obtained from orange blossom flower will hugely be different from that obtained from orange rind as they will come with contrasting properties and hence suitable for therapeutically different benefits. Cashing in on a single essential oil as opposed to pre-mixed remedies or blends is also advisable as: you get to determine the extent of dilution that is suitable for your need, can regulate the nature and intensity of the aroma as well as have a better shelf life since undiluted essential oils last considerably longer.

SHOPPING

Shopping for any material requires due diligence, and essential oils are no exception. With literally endless lists of organic grocery stores, health food stores, cosmetic stores and perfumeries to shop from, ensuring you don't get ripped off takes more than finding a visually appealing website if you decide to purchase online. Getting reliable reviews and samples, if possible, are some ways to nip potential issues in the bud when purchasing an essential oil.

Pricing is another tricky area to consider. You want to compare various outlets for the same product before reaching a decision.

Quality rose otto can be sold anywhere from $300 to $700 per 15ml. There are higher priced alternatives, but you only want to buy those when assured of getting the best value for money. Prices may also hinge on the country of origin, for example, Indian sandalwood essential retails at about $150 per ounce or 30ml, while Australian products from the same sandalwood can be sold for $80 per ounce. Shipping costs may be important too if you are cash-strapped. As some big online outlets can offer free shipping on specific orders, consider that before making a purchase.

Product packaging is equally key. Products packaged in black, brown or dark bottles are especially great since constituents will have been adequately protected from the deteriorating effects of sunlight. The presence of oxygen can also affect the color and odor of essential oils. Stored properly, quality essential oils can last anywhere from 6 to 24 months.

4
WAYS TO USE ESSENTIAL OILS

Essential oils are typically used by topical application or inhalation but never by ingestion, except in extreme cases which should, of course, be guided by a licensed physician or medical personnel.

Inhaling an essential oil helps to balance activities in both right and left parts of the brain. It also stimulates the production and distribution of certain hormones to other parts of the body. When applied topically on the skin, essential oils reach the bloodstream and ultimately get to specific parts of the body that the healing is intended. The specificity of essential oils means they are active and best compatible when in contact with specific hormones, parts of the body, or system. Hence, a product may only work best for muscle tissues, some for bone marrows and so on.

<u>Proper Ways to Apply Essential Oils</u>

Essential oils are typically mild and natural in effect, helping users relieve symptoms of stress, sore muscles, mental fatigue and a host of other conditions. But all these are only possible when applied or used properly. Hence improper use can trigger episodes of allergic reactions and other negative side effects. This is common if, for example, an undiluted essential oil is directly applied to the skin. The result of which may include rash, burn, painful sores or some sort of irritation. A common way to prevent these side effects is to dilute such products in cream or non-greasy oil as may be desired. They should additionally be kept away from the reach of children as they would obviously cause more harm on tender skin when applied undiluted.

Essential oils should be prevented from reaching the eyes, nose or ears as they may cause irritation. If topically applied, wearing latex gloves may help prevent them from becoming excessively absorbed on the fingers. Some essential oils are sensitive to the sun, and so shouldn't be used if you will be going sun tanning afterward. Citrus essential oils are classic examples in this category and include oils like grapefruit oil and bergamot oil.

Testing an essential oil on the skin for any adverse reaction can help in choosing the right product. Simply watch out for any negative effects after dabbing a small quantity on the hand and waiting for 24hrs.

INHALATION METHODS

Inhalation is one of few ways essential oils can be used. Apart from being more convenient and easy to use, it also ensures the potency and effectiveness of the essential oil are not lost when used for aromatherapy. Here are a few ways of inhaling the aroma from essential oils.

- Direct sniffing

This is the fastest and simplest way of inhaling aromas from essential oils. It is done by sniffing from an open vial or wearing a perfume containing the essential oil mixed with a carrier.

- Cupped hands

For a more intense inhalation, a few drops of the oil can be placed on the palm. The hands are cupped over the nose and the oil inhaled by slowly breathing in slowly and exhaling similarly while ensuring that the mouth is closed.

- Diffusion method

In Diffusion, arguably the most thorough inhalation method, oil is diffused into the air using diffusers like electrically heated bowl or candle heated pottery bowl. Other options include a vaporizer, nebulizer, wick inhaler, humidifier, room spray, plug-in atomizer with wick refills, pillow or linen sachet, potpourri or even a multi-reed diffuser. Whichever diffusion method you chose to go with, only a few drops of oil in combination with water or steam will be all that's needed to get the desired therapeutic benefits from essential oils.

TOPICAL APPLICATION

The many ways of topically applying essential oils include:

- Full body massage

Topical application by massaging the full body is the most common way of applying essential oils on the skin. For specific relief from any ailment, the oil massage can be targeted at reflexology points located on the feet and palm soles. The temples are massaged if headache pains are experienced while abdominal problems can be relieved by applying a localized massage to relax muscles involved in digestion.

- Bath water combined with essential oil

A more leisure approach, essential oil-treated bath water or Jacuzzi helps to ease the body and drives home a relaxing feeling after a full body massage.

- By combining with skin products

Another way of topically applying essential oils is by combining your chosen oil with a conditioner, shampoo, face cleanser, moisturizer or lotion. This makes a formidable combination that will both drive a blemish free skin while keeping any inflammatory conditions in check.

DILUTING

In dilution, we mean adding specific drops of essential oil, say three to five drops, to one teaspoon of lotion or carrier oil. This ratio should however be further decreased in the case of facial skin care products. For tub water baths, dissolving in vegetable oil, honey and powdered or liquid milk are reliable ways of ensuring the essential oil is dispersed evenly and not collected in one region.

BLENDING

A best practice is to do your research and have a reliable list of three essential oils that will serve your need. Next is to experiment with them to get the perfect recipe containing the right quantities of your chosen oils before finally combining them for your unique blend. The choice of only three essential oils and a carrier or base oil is to ensure any problems can quickly be identified and fixed immediately. Hence, oils can be removed or added one at a time as you get more acquainted with essential oils. A blend of 5 oils, at most, should suffice for therapeutic use.

5
GENERAL SAFETY PRECAUTIONS

The safety precautions included herein are not exhaustive since essential oils have specific characteristics and so have unique precautions of use. More specific safety precautions of selected essential oils have been provided in the next few chapters. For questions or additional concerns, don't hesitate to consult with your physician or professional aromatherapist.

- The gold standard is to avoid using essential oils directly on the skin when they are "neat" or undiluted. However, tea tree and lavender oils are noticeable exceptions to this rule, but of course, only after experimentation on test patches is successful since some individuals with overly sensitive skin can react to both of these oils, even though they are regarded in aromatherapy as the mildest oils.
- Administration of skin patch test is essential before using an essential oil for the first time.
- Essential oils are not to be used orally, except when advised by, and in the presence of a physician or licensed medical practitioner.
- Essential oils should be used away from fire as they are highly flammable
- If contact is made on sensitive parts like the eye, essential oils should be washed off by irrigation using isotonic, sterile, saline solution for about 15 minutes. Persistent reaction or pains should be reported to a healthcare professional.
- Keep all essential oils away from the reach of children.
- Fennel, rosemary and hyssop are reportedly problematic for patients with epilepsy and so should be avoided if you have

the condition.

- Young babies and the elderly should take lower doses of essential oils since they are negatively reactive to some, especially eucalyptus and peppermint, with respiratory problems commonly reported in users belonging to these age bracket. And as mild as they may appear, only minute quantities, for example, one drop in bath water or ½ drop per ounce of carrier oil of both lavender and neroli is usually tolerated.
- Cancer patients may only use essential oils like chamomile, bergamot, ginger, lavender and frankincense in their mild dilutions, while aniseed and fennel should be avoided.
- Individuals undergoing chemotherapy sessions are advised not to use essential oils to avoid adverse effects.
- Persons with high blood pressure should not use peppermint, black pepper, hyssop, clove, sage, rosemary or thyme essential oils.
- Lavender oil should also be avoided by low blood pressure patients.
- Individuals with the tendency to exhibit allergic reactions to nuts should stay away from peanut or almond carrier oils. Better alternatives to be used instead are canola (non-GM), sunflower and safflower oils.
- Women who are pregnant should stay clear of essential oils prior the 18th week of pregnancy. This is even more important if there is a history of miscarriage. Essential oils may however be used in low doses in the second trimester but should be formulated by an expert aromatherapist or health care professional.

6
TWELVE ESSENTIAL OIL RELAXANTS

BERGAMOT

A predominant citrus fruit grown in Calabria, Italy, Bergamot tastes sour but has a surprisingly lemony, sweet rind with a refreshing and mild fragrance. While it has been grown in parts of the United States and South America, Italian Bergamot leads the pack in all ramifications. The green or yellow oil gotten from bergamot has been extensively used in perfumes and colognes as well as in producing Earl Grey tea where it enhances the unique aroma of the drink. Dubbed the "sunny" oil, bergamot is hugely calming but equally energizing and soothing in effect.

This fruit is effective in treating fever and a wide range of skin conditions like psoriasis, eczema, acne, herpes and oily skin. It also works well for cystitis and many urinary tract infections. While a good appetite stimulant, it also helps in shedding weight.

Bergamot's rich anti-depressant benefits ensure it is a handy regimen for anger, anxiety, stress relief or any Seasonal Affective Disorder (SAD).

PRECAUTIONS:

- Not to be used undiluted on the skin or "neat." Bergamot can be applied on the skin when diluted in a lotion, carrier oil or bath water.
- Bergamot is highly sensitive to the sun, and so should not be used within 12 hours before sun exposure to prevent adverse effects. An exception though is 'Bergaptine Free' or 'Bergamot FCF' labeled bergamot oil which poses no skin problems if used before exposure to the sun.

CHAMOMILE

Extracted from white flowers, Chamomile appears deep blue and tastes sweet and fruity with a subtly bitter undertone. Dried chamomile bearing flowers are commonly used in making chamomile tea which has a positively refreshing aromatic aftereffect. Chamomile comes in different varieties, but Roman and German species are particularly high in medicinal value. Its gentle nature means it is one of very few essential oils that can be used during pregnancy as well as for infants and young children.

Oil from chamomile is a useful anti-inflammatory agent that works effectively against symptoms of allergies like eczema and skin problems like blisters and rash. The analgesic property of chamomile guarantees an invaluable solution for migraines, headaches, stomach ache and premenstrual cramping. Chamomile is also sedative, making it great for anxiety, insomnia, mood swings, nervous tension and other emotional imbalances.

PRECAUTION:

- Fresh chamomile oil appears blue, green colors are signs of deterioration and such should not be used.

CLARY SAGE

This tall herb, also called salvia, comes in purple-green and hairy leaves. When steamed, petals of clary sage give off a musky oil that comes with a nutty tone and enhances mood while being deeply revitalizing and relaxing.

Clary sage oil is analgesic in nature, and so makes it an excellent option for menstrual cramps, stomach pains, hot flashes associated with menopause and pains during labor. It is also effective for headaches and migraines and can be used to relieve asthma too. Dermatologically, applying clary sage can help treat conditions like dandruff for a lush and healthy scalp.

The oil is also known to trigger "high" like properties, therefore making it a strong agent for mood problems like depression and anxiety. It helps stimulate creative thinking, promotes restful sleep and can drive improved meditation.

PRECAUTIONS:

- Being a mood enhancing essential oil, clary sage shouldn't be used with alcohol or other recreational drugs.
- Not suitable for pregnant mothers, young children or individuals 18 years and below.

FRANKINCENSE

Native to African and Middle Eastern Countries and India, Frankincense has a milky-white resin that can be steamed to produce a fresh, woody fragrance essential oil with balsamic, smokey tones. Frankincense has a long history and was synonymously used by a number of religions for purification rites over many centuries. Frankincense oil is known to have a calming and rejuvenating effect and has been used for disinfection and perfume fixative purposes. It has a strong dermal property, thus the essential oil is used in skin care to reverse skin conditions like wrinkles, dry and scaly skin, scars, and stretch marks. Frankincense oil has also been used for bronchitis, asthma, sinusitis, coughing spell, sore throat and cold. The robust essential oil was used in a research at the University of Connecticut in 2008 to successfully treat knee osteoarthritis. Frankincense essential oil is considered strongly effective in helping induce slow deep breathing, quashing feelings of fear and promoting overall emotional strength. Nervous tension, nightmares, sadness, stress and anxiety are other uses of the wondrous Frankincense oil.

LAVENDER

Another beneficial plant used in Aromatherapy is Lavender. Lavender oil is gotten from purple flowers of shrubs with green or gray leaves popularly cultivated worldwide. However, those growing in England and France have particularly been highly appreciated. Lavender oil appears colorless to pale yellow-green and has a characteristic floral fragrance. It is mildly sweet with a woody undertone. Lavender's popularity and widespread use have ensured it is dubbed the "Cure-all Oil" or "Queen of Essential Oils." But it is not hard to see why too. The oil works sublimely effective and blends with essences for improved effectiveness. Lavender oil is considered to stimulate the activation of the brain's pineal gland, thereby helping restore body functions and emotions. It's particularly effective in advancing a calming, relaxing and soothing effect. Lavender is routinely used in the production of skin care products, so expect to find this essential oil in creams and soaps as well as perfumes and household cleaners.

It's considerably mild too; it can be used on infants and young children when diluted in lotions or carrier oils. But that's not all if you fancy adding lavender to your top ten list of essential oils. In combination with massage oil or bath water, Lavender is considered a superb analgesic for muscle spasms and headaches. Viral infections, cold, bronchitis and sinus congestion can also be relieved by using Lavender oil.

The terrific oil can be used undiluted on wound and burn surfaces as it mildly speeds up the healing process. Want to better repel insects or treat their bites? How about allergy induced itching and acne? You can give lavender oil a try for these and more. Lavender is also your reliable oil for anger, mood swings, anxiety, insomnia and hyperactivity while the soothing effect ensures relief is in the offing if you are constantly warding off foggy thinking or want to enhance your insight, rationality and quality of meditation.

PRECAUTION:
- While Lavender oil is undoubtedly beneficial, mothers in the first three months of pregnancy are advised to jettison the use of lavender.

MARJORAM

The bushy herb – Marjoram – has dark silver-green leaves and a bundle of small, whitish pink flowers. Expect a colorless and slightly warm and spicy aroma. Popular uses of Marjoram in Ancient Egypt include perfumes, ointments and flavoring of foods. The essential oil is also called "the great comforter" due to its very powerful sedating benefits.

By dilating the blood vessels, Marjoram finds use in improving circulation and relieving pains including migraine headache, stiff joints, sore muscles, rheumatism and arthritic pains. Digestion problems like flatulence and constipation can also be relieved by taking an abdominal massage session using Marjoram. Stress-induced sexual inactivity can be fixed with this essential oil as it is also an aphrodisiac with a terrific sedating property.

On the emotional end of the spectrum, the oil can help bring back mood downed by grief or loneliness. Insomnia, Obsession (OCD), Hyperactivity (ADD/ADHD) and trauma (PTS) are other conditions that can be reversed by Marjoram oil.

PRECAUTIONS:

- Numbing effects have been reported. Hence, the oil should be used with care. Extended use can cause adverse effects on the senses.
- Not to be used during pregnancy.

<u>NEROLI</u>

Popularly referred to as orange blossoming, Neroli oil, pale yellow in color, comes from the fragrant white flowers of Seville orange. Neroli has a cool floral scent with a characteristically bitter-sweet undertone. It is a popular ingredient used in the production of perfumes and similar cosmetics. A quintessence of purity and innocence, just like its flowers, Neroli is believed to help soothe the evident jitters of a groom or bride. This is due to it's pure, uplifting, calming and slightly hypnotic characteristics. The dazzlingly stunning fragrance is unsurprisingly one of the most expensive essential oils. Neroli oil helps in cell regeneration, so it is a go-to choice for dry and sensitive skin. It helps to tone facial muscles and skin, making it a mainstay in many skin care products and massage oil. Abdominal problems like diarrhea can also be relieved by having a Neroli oil massage.

Professional aromatherapists find this oil top of the list for shock, chronic anxiety and disappointment. Neroli oil is also an effective solution for feelings of despair, depression, hysteria, panic attacks and post-traumatic stress disorder. Rolling back these conditions and enhancing optimism, confidence and initiative driven actions. A mild aphrodisiac, Neroli makes it easier to overcome shyness or anxiety related to sexual activity.

ROSE

Rose is one flower we've all come across. But it's not just its beauty and striking elegance that is captivating. Rose petals are an incredible source of essential that provide numerous benefits. While there are oodles of species of this flower, Damascus, Cabbage or French Rose are exceptionally useful in aromatherapy. A product of water distillation, "Rose otto" is easily the priciest essential oil you can find in the market, selling for around $500 and $1,400 per ounce. You can also cash in on a drop of "Rose otto" between $1.25 to $4.00. The clear to slightly pale yellow oil presents a gentle, light, sweet and spicy aroma. Another option is "Rose Absolute" which distills with alcohol to appear in brown to orange colors with a deep, honeyed aroma that is appreciably stronger than rose otto. In contrast to rose otto, it is not as expensive and can easily be bought at half the price of rose otto. Hence, it is not uncommon to find some aromatherapist prefer rose otto, which they believe is more superior. However, it only comes down to differences in fragrance since the two both have the same therapeutically beneficial properties.

Rose oil finds relevance in many conditions. Like some other essential oils, it is proven beneficial for dry and scaly skin. A massage bath with the oil is also considered particularly effective for women dealing with postpartum depression, premenstrual cramps and menopause. The oil is also an aphrodisiac, and hence can help in reversing sexual anxiety and enhancing confidence instead.

Rose essential oil wards off feelings of sadness, grief or disappointment while fostering a stronger inner spirit. The end result is a comfortable ambiance that radiates inwards and outwards for better expression of love to everyone.

PRECAUTION

- Individuals with a history of miscarriage are advised to stay off this essential oil in the first trimester of pregnancy. However, it can be used without concerns in the second and third trimesters.

SANDALWOOD

The roots and heartwood of sandalwood tree are distilled to get sandalwood oil. The tree itself provides wood that is regarded one of the strongest in the world. Sandalwood essential oil appears pale to dark yellow and has tremendous longevity, staying rich with a radiant fragrance even after an extended period of time when other essential oils would notably have gone rancid.

The oil has a sweet taste with a woody aroma and spicy touch, providing a harmonizing and balancing psyche effect which has ensured its relevance for spiritual use and meditation for thousands of years. The uplifting fragrance has made it a great choice in making male and female perfumes. Indian varieties of sandalwood are widely cherished. The rarity of sandalwood due to growing extinction have driven the high price of this essential oil. However, Australian sandalwood oil can be gotten far cheaper than Indian alternatives and is also considered satisfactorily good by professional aromatherapists.

Essential oil from sandalwood is characteristically calming and soothing and is the most popular option for conditions like laryngitis and bronchitis. The oil is also appreciably effective for urinary tract and bladder infections and has also helped reverse fluid retention. Sandalwood oil has an astringent property, hence it is used for treating a wide range of scalp conditions. When used in bath water of massage oil, sandalwood promotes a relaxing feeling and helps relieve tension and headache. The benefits also encompass aggression, sadness and obsessive thinking. A strong aphrodisiac, the essential oil can be all that's needed to treat stress and depression induced impotence.

PRECAUTION:

- The essential oil is noticeably strong and shouldn't be directly applied on the skin if undiluted.

SPEARMINT

Spearmint essential oil is produced from the distillation of the herb's pink or lilac colored flowers, the leaves of which are luxuriantly green and can grow to about 3 feet long. The oil, yellowish green in color, has a fresh and mint-like aroma that reminds of peppermint. But it is milder and sweeter than the latter.

Suitable for children, the essential oil is a regular flavor in candy, chewing gum, food and medications due to its sweet and cooling effect. The tea from spearmint can be a superb drink when going to bed. It is believed that Ancient Greeks explored the antiseptic and refreshing benefits of spearmint oil by including it in bath water.

A huge range of conditions can benefit from spearmint essential oil. Some of these are chronic respiratory problems including sinusitis and bronchitis. Chest pains and headache can also be relieved using this oil. Other problems that can be treated using spearmint oil are digestive problems synonymous with spams and tension problems. Thus, an abdominal massage can help relieve flatulence, vomiting, hiccups, constipation, and nausea. Its brightening effect means spearmint has found use as a teeth whitener while enhancing gum tissue health. In combination with facial cleansers, this essential oil can help close pores which would otherwise trigger acne, ensuring that your skin is healthier and uniformly toned. Like many other essential oils, spearmint is refreshingly cool and enhances mood, so you can have it a handy inclusion for mild depression and mental fatigue.

PRECAUTIONS:

- While spearmint is usually present in food flavors and common nonprescription medications, it is not a safe practice to ingest any essential oil, including spearmint oil, without due advice and guidance by a medical practitioner.

- In some cases, spearmint can cause irritations in the eyes. It may also be problematic when used on sensitive skin, even if it was diluted before use.

TEA TREE

This shrub has green to yellow leaves that appear needlelike. The tree's bark is characteristically unique and is usually called paper bark due to its papery and white appearance. The essential oil is gotten from the leaves and twigs and has a pungent and spicy aroma like that of nutmeg. The oil is pale yellow and presents a subtle camphor odor. Tea tree is highly active against many infections caused by bacteria, fungi and viruses, hence making it a formidable product in first-aid ointments. The healing and penetrating effects of tea tree oil radiate physically and emotionally. Due to its highly active nature and gentleness, the oil can be applied undiluted on the skin and used to successfully treat conditions including nail fungus, skin rash, cold sores, athlete's foot, herpes, head lice, insect bites, acne and skin abrasions. Discomforting vaginal infection caused by yeast can also be treated by having warm tea tree baths and frequent abdominal massage when combined with a carrier oil.

With gargling and steam inhalation, tea tree oil can help reverse symptoms of sore throat and cold. It can also be used to enhance resistance to sinusitis, bronchitis and laryngitis. The immune system will benefit from the boosting effects of massage and baths with tea tree oil. This is especially advised when suffering from long-term deleterious illnesses like infectious mononucleosis caused by Epstein - Barr virus. Shingles pain can be rescinded by applying Tea tree combined with aloe vera gel. The strong, powerful aroma of tea tree helps to clear the mind, counters fatigue and enhances concentration. By promoting confidence and boosting endurance and strength, Tea tree oil lubricates the mind and positions the body for quicker healing.

PRECAUTIONS:
- Should not be used excessively. Bath water with a maximum of drops is just sufficient. 2% in lotion or massage oil should also not present adverse effects.

- Might have irritating effects, especially when applied on sensitive skin.

YLANG-YLANG

Indonesia is home to the large tropical flowers of the Cananga tree from which the essential oil of ylang-ylang is derived. "ylang-ylang" in Malayan translates as "flower of flowers." The essential oil is clear in appearance, pale yellow in color with an exceedingly sweet, almond fragrance and an exotic, balsamic note. The smell is sensationally captivating and sedating, and hence makes ylang-ylang essential oil a mainstay in perfumes and confectioners. The highest grade of the oil is called "ylang-ylang extra," and is usually first choice for use in aromatherapy.

Although ylang-ylang is used for a good number of conditions, high blood pressure, rapid breathing and unusual heart palpitations are where it is prominently used. Nonetheless, the essential oil is also usually found in skin and hair care products where it is used to treat excessive oiliness. A potent aphrodisiac, an abdominal or groin massage using ylang-ylang can help to reverse frigidity and impotence.

The calming effect makes it a good stress reliever. The essential oil can be used to overcome feelings of anger, frustration, sadness and more intense emotional problems like post-traumatic stress. By helping promote inner tranquillity and peace, ylang-ylang helps conscious meditation and fosters better creative thinking. Adding a few drops of the essential oil in bath water will expectedly enhance mood and relax the mind, both of which are invaluable in treating sleep disorders like insomnia.

PRECAUTIONS:

- To be used only in small amounts. Extensive use over a long period may trigger nausea and headaches. Negative side effects can, however, be prevented by blending ylang-ylang with bergamot or neroli.

7
THE BASIC ESSENTIAL OILS

BASIL

Basil is an aromatic herb with tiny white flowers and yellow-green leaves. Also called "holy basil" or "sweet basil," the essential oil from the herb is pale yellow in color with a sweet, light mint aroma and fruity, spicy fragrance. Basil oil may come across as similar to rosemary oil, but it is noticeably more subtle than the latter. It is mildly stimulating and powers the senses for better stamina. Indians believe the basil herb helps to protect the spirits and homes of inhabitants, hence it is popularly grown in India as a houseplant.

In combination with a massage oil, basil acts a strong anti-spasmodic, helping relieving tensions in the muscle and promoting digestion by relieving digestive spasms. These benefits make the oil of basil a viable product for women experiencing menstrual cramps or chest congestion. Physical exhaustion caused by long-term debilitating illnesses can be remedied using basil oil. Hence it is a perfect springboard when a good burst of energy is needed.

By enhancing quick thinking, basil oil can stimulate better mental awareness and drive good decision making. It is a veritable essential oil for fighting depression, psychic exhaustion or ennui and lethargic feelings. Basil oil also helps to decongest the mind before meditation

PRECAUTIONS:
- Not to be used during pregnancy or by individuals with hypersensitive skin.
- Unsuitable for users under 16.
- Should be used in small quantities not exceeding 2% (6 drops to 1/2 oz) of lotion or carrier oil.

- Extended use and undiluted application can cause adverse effects.

CINNAMON LEAF

Cinnamon essential oil is gotten from leaves of the cinnamon tree. While Cinnamon bark has a strong fragrance and produces a brown/dark-red essential oil, it is peculiarly irritating on the skin, and obviously wouldn't come as first choice for use in aromatherapy. However, cinnamon leaf-derived essential oil is greatly aromatic and has a sweet and spicy fragrance that is slightly peppery and clove-like, except it is sharper and stronger.

Cinnamon is popularly used as a flavor in cooking and also finds huge relevance in medicine. The essential oil obtained from the leaf is inspiring and exhilarating. Cinnamon oil is sublime for cold and bacterial infections when used in a vaporizer or diffuser. It also helps expedites recovery when down with a respiratory illness. Cinnamon, used in abdominal massage, can reverse symptoms of poor digestion, flatulence and flu-like symptoms. The oil is also helpful in relieving stiffness or arthritic pains when used for massage on spines and joints. It can help normalize emotional imbalance, thus it is a great essential oil to quash feelings of sadness and isolation while providing the needed spark for lethargic conditions.

PRECAUTIONS:

- Essential oil of cinnamon leaf should not be used by individuals with sensitive skin.
- Best used in minute quantities. Maximum of 3 drops in bath water, or ½ oz. in lotion or massage oil.

CLOVE BUD

This evergreen is not just popular for producing purple berries and fragrant red flowers; from the center of its blossoms are rose-pink buds that can be dried under the sun and processed by distillation to give the clove essential oil which comes with a fresh and spicy fragrance that mimics cinnamon but different in being less intense or strong.

The oil is pale yellow in appearance and has routinely been an integral part of perfumes, food and medicine for thousands of years in a rich history that dates back to ancient China, Egypt and Rome. The aroma of clove is described as intriguing, mysterious, and mildly stimulating. Clove is therefore a very warming analgesic with a comforting and soothing effect. These benefits mean clove oil provides reliable help in remedying toothache pain when applied on aching tooth or gum tissue. It also works as a breath freshener and works well for muscle ache and joint stiffness that come with arthritis and rheumatism. Indigestion, clove oil enhances appetite and provides solution for indigestion, flatulence and nausea. It is incredibly awesome for illness-induced emotional negativity and generally helps to energize and revitalize the mind for a fulfilling day.

PRECAUTIONS:

- Should not be used on dry or sensitive skin.
- Not to be used excessively to prevent side effects. Bath water should not contain more than three drops of clove oil while massage oil and lotions are best combined with ½ ounce of the oil.

EUCALYPTUS

Eucalyptus is extremely diverse with more than seven hundred species known. However, only about twenty of these are important in aromatherapy, with each having slight differences. The evergreen eucalyptus tree can grow as high as 30 meters, producing dark green leaves wherefrom the essential oil is obtained. The oil has a characteristically sharp aroma, with a woody and balsamic tone. Eucalyptus is widely invigorating and piercing and is among a few essential oils with a consistently increasing potency as it ages. Eucalyptus is easily a go-to choice when treating colds, sinusitis or bronchitis, regardless of if it's a viral, bacterial or fungal infection. It can be used via steam inhalation to clear respiratory problems while treating headache, sore throat and neuralgia.

Being a potent essential oil against bacteria, it is used as a deodorizer and disinfectant in rooms when in a diffuser or vaporizer. Eucalyptus essential oil is also a great insect repellant and works well in treating insect bites. In bath water, the oil can reverse symptoms of rashes and shingles, while blending with bergamot is an effective solution for cold sores and herpes.

The invigorating and purifying feature means it takes away emotional and mental exhaustion successfully. "lemon eucalyptus" presents a powerful fragrance that can help promote mental agility and concentration during tasks and also helps to clear the mind, allowing for effective sessions when meditating or praying.

GERANIUM

No essential oil can be gotten from ornamental garden geranium. Additionally, only one out of over seven hundred known geranium varieties is relevant in aromatherapy. The whole geranium plant including the stalls, hairy serrated leaves, pink to magenta or red clusters of florets are needed to obtain an essential oil, the fragrance of which is lemon like and herbal with a reminiscent of rose. The light green essential oil is however cheaper than rose oil and is often present in perfumes to make rose oil more effective. The oil has an aroma that provides a harmonizing, refreshing and uplifting effect while fueling increased sense of stability and security.

By stimulating the adrenal cortex, geranium is known to help reverse hormonal imbalance that may present varying problems in women with menopausal symptoms and menstrual cramps. Geranium also has an antiseptic property that makes it invaluable for lymph detoxification or aiding minor wounds in the flesh. It's beautification effects is hinged on regulating skin glands and stalling overproduction of oil, both of which are actively problematic, causing acne and other skin problems.

Geranium helps to promote better circulation that can be helpful in the optimal functioning of the urinary system. Used in massage oil, geranium can be routinely used to reduce cellulite. It can help repel insects and works effectively as a room freshener. Germanium oil in considerably emotionally beneficially and helps to ward off depression, mood swings, anxiety and nervousness as well as stress and fatigue.

JASMINE

A flowering shrub, Jasmine has nice green leaves and white blossoms from which the essential oil is derived by solvent extraction to give a "Jasmine absolute" – the only form of jasmine essential oil. The dark orange colored oil has a strong fragrance with a sweet, honey undertone. But it does take a lot of jasmine flowers to produce a decent amount of Jasmine absolute. About one thousand pounds of jasmine flowers yield less than 4.5 grams of the absolute. So, it is understandably one of the most expensive oils on the market. Jasmine gives off its strongest scent at night, and hence it is popularly dubbed the "queen of the night." The oil is mildly hypnotic but surely euphoric, liberating, and assuredly revitalizing. Little wonder it goes as a first choice perfume for many users.

But that's not all there is about Jasmine. Apart from scenting well and holding strong in perfumes, it also works excellently in the skin department by helping rejuvenate and giving a vibrant look. Added to warm water, Jasmine absolute can be used to effectively combat joint stiffness, muscle spasm and sustained episodes of sprained ligaments. It's also reproductively beneficial for both gender, as it can be used in back or abdominal massage to reduce labor pains and reduce discomforts that may occur when the prostate gland becomes enlarged. A strong aphrodisiac effect positions it to help stir vigor and stimulate passions for a happier family.

The solidly stimulating nature makes it a reliable antidepressant that can bring back the confidence and good sense of judgment needed for individuals dealing with lethargy and indecision problems. Hence, it thwarts pessimism, annihilates fear and rules out paranoia, the end result being a more rounded and elevated thinking with enhanced positive emotions.

LEMON

The rind of lemon fruit produces the essential oil when cold pressed. Lemon essential oil appears yellowish green but differs from that of "lemon-petitgrain," "lemon balm" or "lemongrass," all of which have different aromatherapy benefits due to their characteristic properties. Lemon oil gives off a sweet scent that reminds of fresh lemon rind, however, it is stronger and longer lasting. Lemon oil is often present perfume, personal care products as well as in household cleaners. It also has relevance in medicine and is a popular addition in food flavoring. Lemon oil comes with a refreshing, invigoration and purifying aroma.

The essential oil is ideal for use in detoxifying all of the respiratory, circulatory and lymphatic systems. It is also a good wound cleanser and can be used to treat sore throat and colds due to its antibacterial properties. An acid neutralizer, lemon oil is additionally great for gout and neutralizes excessively acidic stomach. It can as well be used for rheumatism. Included in skin care products, lemon works to reverse dull and oily skin, while clearing dark spots and varicose veins. Used in addition to shampoo or to rinse hair after a wash, lemon is known to enhance a crisp and dazzling sheen. Bathing in lemon oil can aid recovery from mental fatigue or help to regain vigor after sustained exhaustion from physical activity. Lemon oil enhances fast decision making and rids the mind of anything that impedes concentration, thereby making it an ideal use before mediation.

PRECAUTIONS:

- Lemon oil is particularly sensitive to light, and so should not be applied 24hours before sun exposure
- To be avoided by individuals with sensitive skin.
- Should be used minimally. Not more than three drops in bath water. Massage oil or lotion should not contain more than ½ ounce of lemon oil.

PATCHOULI

Leaves of Patchouli are large, hair and soft. To get Patchouli essential oil, the leaves are first dried and subsequently fermented for a number of days before distillation. This ends with the production of dark orange essential oil whose fragrance is characteristically spicy and wood, with a smoky and balsamic presence. A strong agent used in perfumes, patchouli is also a good deodorizer and also employed to repel moth in carpeting and woven fabrics. The oil is aphrodisiac too, and so both balances and rejuvenates sensual vigor.

A number of skin anomalies can be reversed by applying patchouli essential oil. Some of these conditions include oily skin, dermatitis, dandruff and athlete foot. It particularly helps in skin renewal and helps conceal scar with its regenerative properties.

A great insect repellant, patchouli oil can be useful in treating snake bites too. The essential oil can help deal with pertinent sexual problems including male impotence and frigidity in females.

The emotional benefits make it excellent for anxiety, anger, nervousness and other emotional imbalances. Negative thoughts can ignite depressive moods and confusion can lead to extended vacillation and procrastination, however, they can also be effectively reversed by Patchouli. It is also used to remedy episodic daydreaming and withdrawal problems from hard drugs like tobacco.

PEPPERMINT

The peppermint plant produces flowering tops and downy leaves from which the famous peppermint oil is distilled. The oil is virtually colorless and has a fresh and penetrating smell. The history of peppermint dates back to thousands of years ago when it was popularly explored in ancient Greece and Egypt. This hasn't affected its distribution today, though, as it has gained massive popularity the world over, and is commonly used in food flavoring, candy, gum and in nonprescription drugs. The characteristic pungent aroma comes from menthol, which is predominantly present in amounts ranging from 50% to 80%. Peppermint is highly refreshing, energizing and gives a soothing feel. It has been widely used to help relieve headaches due to its analgesic properties.

A number of digestive problems also respond well to abdominal massage with peppermint oil. Some of these conditions include diarrhea, irritable bowel syndrome, constipation, flatulence, motion sickness, colon spasm and nausea. Carrier oil dilution and application on forehead, temples and neck can help douse migraine pains. Arthritic pains, leg spasm, muscle ache and menstrual cramps can as well be improved with a peppermint massage.

The essential oil can be used as an expectorant or decongestant by massaging on the chest to relieve bronchitis, colds, cough, asthma and sinusitis. Peppermint oil is also reliably antiviral, helping clear herpes and influenza. Fungal yeast and athlete foot infections can also benefit from Peppermint oil. When used as an antiseptic, the essential oil can work to prevent tooth decay, bad breath and gum disease. Inhaled peppermint oil enhances alertness, improves mental clarity and ensures concentration is at its peak. Hence, peppermint fights mental fatigue as well as feelings of apathy and insecurity.

PRECAUTIONS:
- Allergic reactions might be experienced when used on sensitive skin. Thus, it should never be used neat, but in combination with a lotion, carrier oil or bath water.
- Peppermint should not be used for children aged less than five years as chances of adverse reactions to menthol is likely.

<u>PINE NEEDLE</u>

Scotch pine may be popularly recognized by its unique red bark, it also has cones, branches and needle-like leaves from which its essential oil is derived. The pine needles are however the most preferred source for producing the essential oil for aromatherapy use. The clear oil produced smells fresh, with a balsamic fragrance and subtle feel of turpentine. The oil derived from pine has been hugely included in cleansers, soaps, and deodorants alike due to its strong antiseptic properties. A sauna bath ensures its energizing and invigorating effects are fully derived.

The essential oil is the most ideal for making lungs phlegm free. It also has additional respiratory benefits that make it ideal for conditions like sinusitis, colds, hay fever and bronchitis. It is strong against a host of other viral and bacterial infections. In vaporizer, pine oil can bring breathing relief asthma patients while disinfecting the air too.

In massage lotion, pine oil can help treat injuries developed from sports like muscle strain due to excessive exertion and sprains. Bathing with pine oil is believed to help clear cystitis and also gently stimulate and revive weak bladder or kidney function by providing diuretic benefits. It is also a worthy inclusion when treating cellulite with massage.

Pine essential oil helps to relieve symptoms of fatigue as well as mental exhaustion occasioned by tension and irritability. An air diffusion of pine oil brings an aura of confidence, forgiveness and takes away guilt feelings, providing an improved ambiance suitable for meditation.

PRECAUTION:

- Can cause skin irritation even when diluted, especially on individuals with sensitive skin.

ROSEMARY

Essential oil can be derived from the blue flowers of the Rosemary shrub. The resulting colorless and thin oil presents a herbaceous aroma with a tinge of camphor and balsam, ensuring that rosemary has a fresh, medicinal odor. Rosemary is historically considered to help create a form or protection against negative energy and emotions. Consequently, it is used in funerals and weddings for this purpose. It is however commercially used in the preparation of skin care products.

As with all essential oils, loads of benefits abound using rosemary oil. For starters, few drops of the oil can be added in conditioner, shampoo or rinse water to help better stimulation of the scalp, and thus helps to keep off dandruff and promote stronger and better hair growth. In facials, rosemary oil is characteristically revitalizing and rejuvenating, ensuring that dull skin is quickly brought back to life. Going for a full body massage with rosemary oil will help stimulate improved circulation and controlled stiffening on the joints, thereby fighting muscle aches, neuralgia, spasm, arthritis, gout and rheumatism.

The oil is great for use in preventing airborne infection when diffused into the air. Rosemary is considered the foremost essential oil when looking to maintain and improve brain function as it enhances mental stability, increases emotional strength and helps to recover from emotional stress, confusion and general negativity usually experienced with a poor mental balance. It also enhances memory and thus easily tops the chart for students and writers as it helps better intuitive vision, enhances creative thinking and declutters the mind of any impediment to free-flowing mental energy. Rosemary oil is also considered to aid practical thinking and facilitates a better approach when solving emotional, physical and spiritual problems. It is another invaluable essential to fully focus the mind before going on meditation.

PRECAUTION:

- Not to be used during pregnancy or by patients suffering from fever or epilepsy

THYME

Essential oil of this bushy shrub is extracted from its leaves and white top flowers. Over 150 species of thyme are known, the most powerful of which is "red thyme" that has a brown-red or orange color. Red thyme is best applied for use in aromatherapy by air diffusion as it has a high phenol concentration which could cause skin irritation if used otherwise. However, there is subtler variety in "thyme linalool" which is a thin, pale yellow liquid that can be used on the skin after diluting in a bath water or carrier oil.

A multi-distillation of red thyme called "white thyme essential oil" can be purchased from some manufacturers and is regarded to be more skin friendly.

Whichever the variety, all thyme varieties seem to have identical smells with red thyme being particularly most pungent. Red thyme also has a sweet, spicy and subtly medicinal aroma. Oil from thyme was chiefly used in ancient civilizations of Rome, Egypt and Greece. The oil was essentially used in baths, massage oil, burners, disinfectant and general atmospheric fragrance due to its purifying, energizing, re-balancing and strengthening characteristics.

Thyme oil is also important in fighting bacterial and viral infection. Additionally, it stimulates white blood cells production and consequently makes the immune system more resistant to infections, preventing it from sore throat, colds and influenza.

By enhancing production of red blood cells, thyme oil ensures oxygen is distributed faster to all parts of the body, thereby making the body refreshed and reinvigorated. The oil is helpful in enhancing appetite which usually dips in individuals who are ill. Thyme oil is used to aid digestion and solve constipation problems. The ripple effect is a terrifically energized body and a strongly balanced system. Lost stamina due to fatigue and male impotence and sexual frigidity can all be reversed too.

PRECAUTIONS:

- Thyme has many varieties, however, they shouldn't all be used during pregnancy and also by individuals who have problems with high blood pressure.
- Red thyme should not be used in any case as a massage oil or added in bath water. It is also best avoided for children.

With that, we have come to the end of this book. I want to thank you for choosing this book.

Now that you have come to the end of this book, we would first like to express our gratitude for choosing this particular source and taking the time to read through it. All the information here was well researched and put together in a way to help you understand the essential oils as easily as possible.

We hope you found it useful and you can now use it as a guide anytime you want. You may also want to recommend it to any family or friends that you think might find it useful as well.

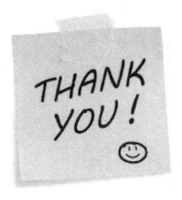

Printed in the USA
CPSIA information can be obtained
at www.ICGtesting.com
LVHW041030310124
770323LV00008B/124